THE ULTIMATE EXERCISE

Awesome Golden exercises as recommended by a physical therapist for physical and mental health wellbeing

Jordan Chris

copyright@2021

Table of contents

CHAPTER ONE

   WHAT ARE ULTIMATE EXERCISES?

CHAPTER TWO

   10 Golden Full Body Exercises

   1. Burpees

   2. Squats

   3. Step ups

   4. Pull ups

5. Push ups

   6. Dips

   7. Jump lunges

   8. Kettlebell swings

   9. Handstands

   10. Box Jumps

CHAPTER ONE

WHAT ARE ULTIMATE EXERCISES?

With regards to working out, a large portion of us would like to get most extreme outcomes in the briefest measure of time conceivable.

So it doesn't really make so much sense when individuals invest the entirety of their energy in the rec center on single muscle isolation exercises like biceps twists or curls, extension of legs and triceps kickbacks when they could be getting more stronger, quicker and consume more calories in less time with full body works out.

While isolation exercises are incredible for weight lifters attempting to acquire gigantic size, they're not really the most productive activities or the most ideal decision for the regular exerciser hoping to get in the best shape in a restricted measure of time.

Besides the fact that full body exercises makes one functionally fit i.e it will help you perform excellently well in your day to day activities, they are also known to function by working additional muscles at one time and consume extra calories in the process of doing it.

I have put together 10 full body exercises that will cause you to be more fit and healthier both physically and mentally.

CHAPTER TWO

10 Golden Full Body Exercises

1. Burpees

In the event that I needed to pick my number one exercise ever, burpees would be it. Not exclusively do burpees require only your own bodyweight—which means you have no genuine reason not to do them—they're a marvelous by and large body strengthener and will condition you like no other exercise can.

How to do carry out burpees:

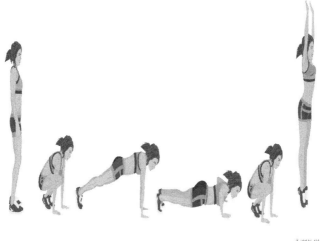

Stand upright, at that point get into a squat situation with your hands on the floor before you. Kick your feet back into a push up position and lower your body with the goal that your chest contacts the floor. Then jump and return your feet to the squat situation as quick as could reasonably be expected. Promptly jump up as high as could be expected under the circumstances. Add a little applauds.

You have done well!!!

2. Squats

Not exclusively will squats give you a solid, amazing lower body, they'll additionally work your center, reinforce your back and your shoulders also.

Besides, you can do squats utilizing only your own body weight for a magnificent, do-anyplace work out, add weight to make them considerably all the more testing.

How to carry out Squats:

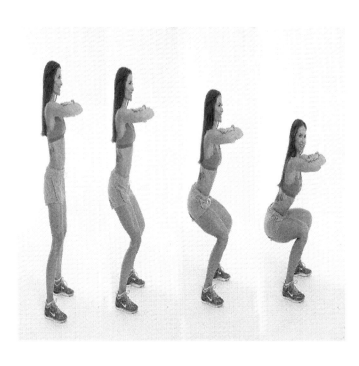

Stand with your feed hip-width separated while pulling your shoulders back and drawing in your abs. Push your butt and hips back as though you were sitting in a seat. While keeping your weight behind you, drop down until your thighs are equal or lower to the floor. Raise back up to the beginning position, pressing your butt and pushing your knees outward as you straighten.

3. Step ups

Step ups are a fabulous exercise you can do with next to no space that will reinforce your legs and center muscles, build endurance, and get the rate of your heart up and all this can be achieved in a single move.

To make step ups all the more testing, add weight or step onto a higher surface.

How to carry out step ups:

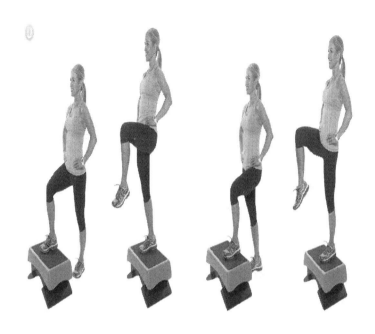

Stand before a container or a raised surface, pulling your shoulders back and keeping your abs tight. Set your left leg onto the container, at that point step to top of the case ensuring your feet are level. Step down with a similar leg, at that point rehash with your right leg.

4. Pull ups

Pull ups are outstanding amongst several upper body exercises, it not only work on your arms, back and shoulders, it also helps to reinforce or strengthen your core. In the event that you can't do one yet, don't surrender all expectation—with training, anybody can do a draw up (truly, that incorporates ladies!).

How to perform pull ups:

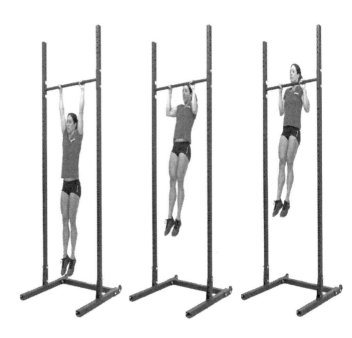

Start by dangling from a pull up bar with your palms turning away from you. Keeping your chest up and your shoulders back, press your glutes and cross your feet, at that point pull yourself up so your jawline rests over the bar. Let back down wlth ſull control.

Pull up modifications for beginners:

•	**Jumping pull ups:** Jump up from the beginning a raised surface, utilizing energy to help drive yourself up to the bar.

•	**Negatives:** Jump up to the bar so that you're in the highest point of a draw up position, at that point gradually drop yourself down with control.

•	**Use bands:** Looping a band around the draw up bar and afterward again around your feet (or knees) can help you push past the staying purpose of the draw up.

5. Push ups

Disregard the extravagant machines, do push ups all things considered. Pushups work your arms, back, chest, center, butt and even leg muscles. What's more, the best thing about pushups? You can do them anyplace.

How to carry them out:

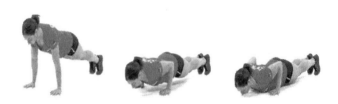

Start in a plank position, with your shoulders straightforwardly over your hands. Make your abs tight, glutes and thighs, at that point drop yourself down so your chest contacts the floor while keeping your elbows as near your body as could be expected under the circumstances. Propel yourself back up into the beginning position and repeat the process.

Push ups modifications for starters:

•   **Incline push ups:** Find a seat, a table, or a comparative solid raised surface and accept a plank position with your feet on the floor and your hands on the raised surface. Do a push up from this position. As you get more grounded, discover lower surfaces to do them on.

•   Push ups from your knees: Start in a push up situation with your knees on the floor. Fix your abs, glutes and thighs, at that point drop yourself down so your chest contacts the floor while keeping your elbows as near your body as could reasonably be expected. Propel yourself back up into the beginning position and replicate the process.

6. Dips

Need to work your chest or triceps, rear arm muscles, shoulders and abs at the same time? Begin making dips your go-to work out.

The most effective method to do them:

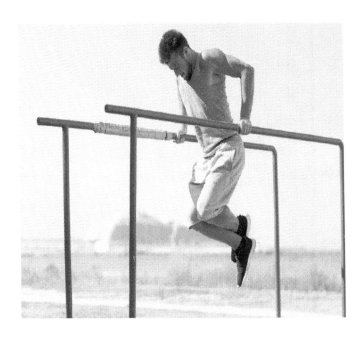

Stand in the middle of parallel bars. Get a hold on the bars, fix your arms, and lift yourself up off the ground while marginally folding your legs. While pulling your shoulders back and keeping your chest up, drop yourself down with the goal that your elbows are corresponding to the floor. Raise yourself back up to the beginning position with the goal that your arms are straight.

Dips modifications for beginners:

- **Elevate your feet:** Assume similar position between a set of parallel bars as portrayed above, however put your feet on a raised surface to make it simpler.

- **Use a bench:** Sit on a seat or tough surface with your feet on the floor and your hands behind you, elbows bowed behind you. Raise yourself up off the seat with the goal that your arms are straight feet still on the ground. While holding your shoulders back and abs tight, bring down your butt to the seat, so your elbows structure a 90 degree point. Raise yourself back up and replicate the process.

7. Jump lunges

Jump lunges won't just cause your legs to burn like something else, they'll get your heart rate up rapidly also and challenge your skills that concerns balancing—making them a fabulous whole body conditioning exercise.

Instructions on how to do them:

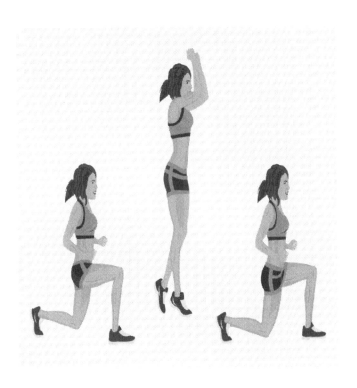

Start in a lunge spot with your knees contacting or practically contacting the floor. And then explosively jump up and switch legs so your back leg is in the front and your front leg goes to the rear leg, at that point replicate the process as quick as possible.

8. Kettlebell swings

Everybody from body builders to the normal lover of exercise loves kettlebell swings for a good reason: they rock. Not exclusively are kettlebell swings incredible for fat reduction, they'll build power increase, boost muscular endurance, also have the ability to increase your aerobic and anaerobic activities and much more.

How to do them:

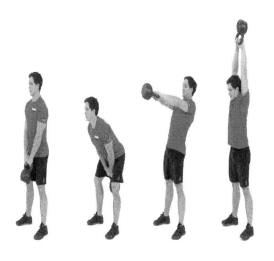

Stand with your legs hip-width separated, holding a portable weight between them. Permit the portable weight to swing somewhat behind your legs, at that point push your hips forward, bringing the iron weight straight over your head. Keep your eyes on the portable weight and point it straight up or marginally forward. Pull the portable weight down from the sky and rehash.

9. Handstands

Handstands are perhaps the most underestimated exercises for one fundamental explanation: the vast majority think they can't do them. In any case, regardless of whether you begin doing handstands against a wall, they'll help you acquire a strong chest area and core, boost your balancing capacities, help in bone wellbeing, and much more.

Truth be told, doing handstands consistently can even assistance you feel less worried and believe everyone need rest of mind and reduced stress.

How to do them:

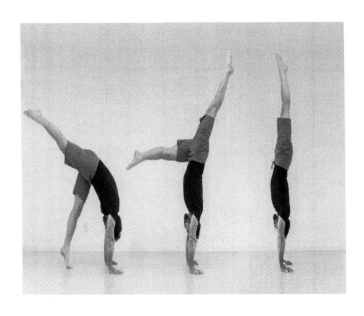

Start with your hands on the ground in a region where there's nothing around you to bump upon. Tuck or jump up with control and hold the handstand. Drop yourself down with control.

Handstand modifications for starters:

- **Handstand facing away from the wall**: Face away from the wall with your hands on the ground shoulder width separated.

- Slowly walk your feet up the wall until you're vertical, at that point walk your hands near the wall. Escape the handstand by strolling your feet down. Attempt to hold a handstand for 5-10 seconds for six sets. On the off chance that this is excessively extreme for you actually, work on strolling here and there the wall until you develop enough strength.

- **Handstand confronting the wall:** Face toward the wall,

place your hands on the ground shoulder width separated, and hop up into a handstand with control. Work up to holding a handstand for 60 seconds. Whenever you have that down, then try your best to remove your feet from the wall.

10. Box Jumps

Extraordinary for developing lower body strength, conditions and prepares your body for any sporting activities that involves jumping, box jumps additionally consume significant calories and will get your pulse up in a rush.

Besides, bouncing up on something high makes you resemble a boss, and who doesn't need that?

How to do carry out Box jumps:

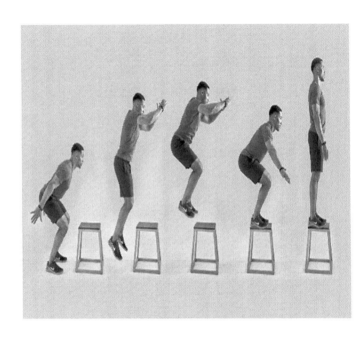

Stand before a box or solid raised surface. Jump up onto the box, arrival with both of your feet on top at that point fix your legs. Jump down from the box, at that point promptly hop back up and do it once more.

Now go ahead and get to work, get sweaty, and have fun and live a healthy life!

Made in the USA
Monee, IL
16 October 2022

16016844R00022